M000040443

This Notebook Belongs To
